*Development of this guidebook was
made possible through a grant from
the* **Meyer Memorial Trust.**

We would also like to thank
Western Graphics & Data
for printing services.

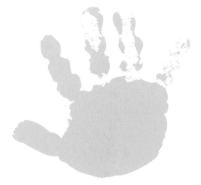

The Dougy Center for
Grieving Children
3909 S.E. 52nd Avenue
P.O. Box 86852
Portland, OR 97286

Voice: 503•775•5683

Fax: 503•777•3097

E-mail: help@dougy.org

Website:
www.dougy.org

Written and printed in
the United States of
America.

ISBN: 1-890534-05-6

When Death Impacts Your School

Table of Contents

This guidebook was developed by The Dougy Center, The National Center for Grieving Children & Families. Since 1982, the Center has worked with thousands of children, teens and their adult family members who have experienced the death of a parent, adult caregiver, sibling or teen friend.

At The Dougy Center, we are often called upon to help a school community cope after a death. We have provided assistance to principals, counselors, teachers and other staff in hundreds of schools following a death. During these interventions, we teach the faculty what to expect from grieving students and staff, as well as ways to support them. Frequently, we also meet with students, parents, and families who are directly impacted by a death to discuss their needs and concerns. We have found that when school personnel address the death directly, talk openly about their concerns, allow grieving, and plan memorials, they are better able to facilitate healing and help students move forward constructively.

In an earlier guidebook, "Helping the Grieving Student: A Guidebook for Teachers," we shared information and practical suggestions about how to help students through the grieving process in the classroom. Drawing from our experiences working with schools, we have created this companion guidebook for school principals who come in direct contact with students and faculty who are grieving a death.

In times of crisis, we look for leaders to guide us. Strong leadership gives people the sense of security they need to begin the healing process. As a principal, you have the unique and sometimes daunting privilege of sharing in the joys and tragedies of students' and teachers' lives. We hope that the information presented here will equip you with the necessary skills to lead effectively and sensitively when a death occurs in your community.

We dedicate this book to the thousands of children, teens, and adults who have courageously shared their pain, their stories, and their healing. They, the grievers, have been our best teachers and leaders at The Dougy Center.

The Principal's Role in Helping Grieving Students and Staff

It was the night before Thanksgiving. The Moore family was getting ready to go to a church service. Lydia Moore went upstairs to check on her 11-year-old son, who had been in a time-out. What she saw when she entered the room made her scream. Using shoelaces tied together, Jake had hung himself in his closet. Lydia and her husband, and later paramedics, tried unsuccessfully to revive him. Within the hour, the Moore's firstborn, their only son, was dead.

In the midst of the shock and numbness that engulfed her in the early days after her son died, Lydia had an important realization: she was not the only one grieving. She thought a lot about her daughters, her son's friends and classmates, and his teachers. What could be done for them? What would Jake want? All of sudden, it was very clear to her what she needed to do: go to her children's elementary school and talk about what happened with the school community. As difficult as it was, this visit was

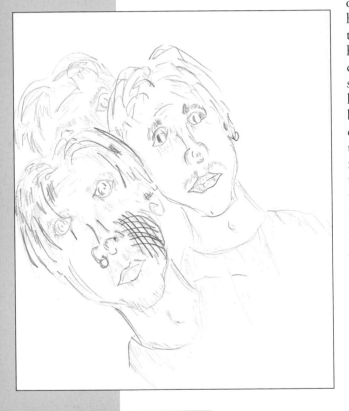

one of the most helpful and healing things Lydia did for herself, her daughters and her son's friends. "I knew I had to go because these children had a grief to bear," she recalled. "I wanted to tell them the truth, and not have them hear it second hand. It was hard, but I had to do it." While in the classrooms, Lydia talked openly with her son's friends and classmates and answered their questions about the death.

An important ally during this time was Lydia's school principal. Immediately after the death, the principal contacted all of the parents in both her son's and her daughters' classrooms. This helped ensure that the children received accurate information about the death before they came to school, and had a chance to talk with their parents. The principal also provided a safe setting in which students and staff could discuss the death. He made a way for children to mourn the death of their friend Jake, and helped Lydia's daughters feel accepted and loved at a time when they felt different from other children. In later years, the principal continued to honor Jake by memorializing him with a plaque in a picnic area by the playground. "He handled the situation properly and with the greatest sensitivity," Lydia said.

Of course, not all parents would choose—nor would it be advisable in all situations—to handle a death in the unique and up front way Lydia did. What is important about Lydia's story is the way in which her son's principal intervened to help facilitate a healing process for the family, faculty, and other students who were affected by the death.

When a death occurs, whether it is from a suicide like Jake's, an accident, an illness, or an act of violence, the entire school community is impacted. In a very difficult and tumultuous time, Lydia's principal played a strong leadership role in the grief process of the family and the school community. How he handled the situation set the stage for the healing process for everyone affected by the death. Although every family and every situation is unique, what really made a difference for the Moores, and for many other families who have experienced a death, is that the school principal and staff were prepared, pro-active, and sensitive in their responses to a significant loss.

The Importance of Having a Plan

We are rarely ready for the impact of the death of someone close to us. However, we can prepare in advance to respond sensitively to the community of grievers affected by a loss. It would be unthinkable for a school not to have a fire escape plan or "lock down" plan in case of an emergency. Nonetheless, many schools do not have a "crisis intervention" plan that includes a response strategy for the death of a student, faculty member or friend.

As a society, we are uncomfortable talking openly about death and grief. We'd much rather sweep those painful, awkward feelings and thoughts under the rug and move on. We'd also like to protect ourselves and our children from pain. We fear that by bringing up the death, we will make it worse for children. Usually, it's just the opposite. If you cover an open wound and leave it unattended, it will not heal properly. By the same token, if you act as though grief doesn't exist just because people aren't talking about it, more often than not it will show up in unwanted behaviors or emotional problems later.

With recent incidences of violence on school campuses, there has been a shift in the way educators and students think about safety. People are more aware that they need to be prepared for the possibility of a violent event and its aftermath. But there is still a lot of misinformation and confusion about what to do with our grief after a person dies. Should we talk about it? Do we need counseling for it? When do we "get over" it? In reality, your school is a lot more likely to experience the death of an individual than a violent incident with multiple deaths. Either way, our attitude toward death should be the same: Hope it doesn't happen, but make a plan for dealing with it when it does.

Elements of the Plan

In any crisis situation, it's difficult to remember everything that needs to be accomplished. Often there are many fires to put out, decisions to be made, help to be found. In the midst of the chaos, how do you find time to speak with the concerned parent on the phone?

To comfort your staff? To advise the troubled teen in your office? When you have a response plan, you and your staff can anticipate what you might need to do in a crisis in advance, and can lay out strategy to handle a situation in a smooth, orderly and sensitive way. Then, when the crisis hits, you have immediate access to resources that will help staff and students. The response plan is general in nature, and can be adapted to any situation. Your school may need to establish policies that deal with media, use of consultants, funeral attendance, and memorial activities. Each plan should cover these basic areas:

- How to set up a Crisis Response Team
- How to respond to a death in the school community
- An outline of the first school day/week following a death
- A long-term plan after the death
- Staff training regarding implementation of the plan
- Information about dealing with grief and death with students
- Informing and dealing with parents
- Ways to communicate effectively with the media
- Memorialization activities
- Continuation of services beyond the crisis time

Setting up a Crisis Response Team

The Crisis Response Team is your greatest asset during the initial period following a death. The team's role is to collect necessary information, help contact and support other staff members, and implement the intervention plan.

Who is on the Team?

Typically, a team consists of 4-8 members with each member making a commitment of one or two years. Team members could include teachers, counselors, administrators, secretaries, parents, custodians, coaches, kitchen staff, bus drivers, and/or other support staff.

Responding to a Death in Your School

Roles of Team Members

Assign general roles and areas of responsibilities to team members prior to a crisis. A team should have a liaison to each of the following groups: parents, local media, police and community mental health resources. Each of these liaisons can gather information and make contacts for use following a death. For example, the media liaison might contact a reporter on the education beat of a local newspaper. On the educational front, one or more team members can be assigned to organize 1) training for team and staff, 2) providing curriculum on death and dying, grief, suicide prevention and other related topics, 3) assembling a community resource list for the team. All educational and resource materials should be reviewed and approved by the committee before use.

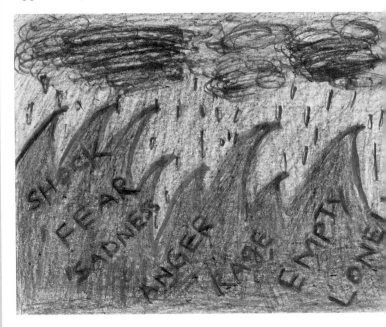

It is important to note that roles of team members will not necessarily be the same during a crisis. For example, if a student's mother dies of cancer, a media or police liaison would not be necessary. Specific roles at the time of the death may also change if a member of the team is ill, personally impacted by the death, or is unable to fulfill his or her responsibilities for some other reason.

Training for the Team

It will be important for you and your team members to educate yourselves in a variety of areas including:

- Working with people who are traumatized
- Understanding developmental issues of grief
- Supporting grieving students/faculty
- Identifying and referring at-risk children

You may want to utilize resources in your community for training. Professionals from a local hospice or bereavement support programs may be of help, as well as your own counseling staff.

The Tasks of the Team Before a Crisis

Some of the most important work of the Crisis Response Team should occur in anticipation of a crisis or death. The completion of certain tasks reduces the level of confusion and chaos that is often an aspect of an unexpected death, and equips the team to respond with the greatest efficiency and sensitivity when a death occurs. Here is a checklist of general tasks to be completed by the team:

☐ Establish a written plan and policy for responding to a death in your school

☐ Write policy for areas including media, memorials, funeral attendance

☐ Develop training for the team and other faculty

☐ Review the plan annually and assign responsibilities

☐ Create a communication "tree" to inform all parties of the crisis, keep it up to date

☐ Assign roles of team members (e.g., liaisons to media, police, family)

☐ Determine a plan for the flow of information

☐ Develop a written statement that can be used by teachers to inform students about the death
(See Appendix A)

- [ ] Develop a handout for teachers on common grief responses, behaviors to expect, and what to do when there is a problem

- [ ] Write a letter to parents to be sent home at the end of the day (or to be mailed) *(See Appendix B)*

The Tasks of the Team During a Crisis

When a death occurs, the Crisis Response Team needs to meet as soon as possible. This may be after school hours or during weekend or vacation days. If the death occurs during non-school hours, it is important that there is an action plan in place when students return. If the death occurs during the school day, it's best that the team meets immediately. The action plan covers five basic task areas:

- Confirm the Death

- Inform Staff, Students and Parents About the Death

- Plan Schedules and Activities for the School Day and Week

- Provide Safety Measures and Special Services for Students

- Assign Jobs and Roles to Crisis Response Team Members

Confirm the Death

As the principal, you need to personally confirm that the death has actually occurred. Do not rely on potentially inaccurate information such as hearsay or even media reports. This is a matter of your reputation and leadership. You need to be informed so you can lead your staff and students through the crisis. All staff and students should be aware in advance that any information they receive about a death should be passed on to you immediately.

Next, you need to confirm the information about the death, or appoint someone from the team to get accurate information. Don't underestimate how important it may be for some families to have you (and not another staff member) call them. Getting accurate information may involve speaking to law enforcement and/or a family member about what happened, and gathering as much detail as possible about the circumstances, time and cause of the death. Any information about what has happened needs to be verified before you share it with students and staff. This helps prevent rumors and inaccurate information from being spread.

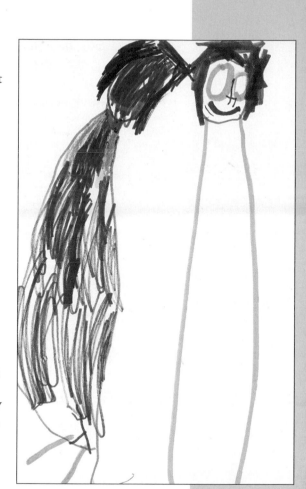

As you talk with family members, review specifically what information will be shared with school personnel and students and how you plan to go about this. If possible, include the family in planning what is shared, respecting their privacy, while informing them of the importance of sharing accurate information with the faculty and students. Sometimes, families will not want information shared with students. You may have to work with them to understand the importance of truth-telling. Although it is not necessary to share all the details of a death, you can emphasize to families that children in particular will be seeking answers and trying to find out the truth any way they can. If they are not told, more often than not, they come up with stories which are more fantastic than the truth. These stories may be hurtful to friends, family and siblings of the deceased. You may also want to discuss with the family details about memorial or funeral services, and find out how they feel about school personnel and students attending such events.

Inform Staff, Students and Parents About the Death

In the aftermath of a crisis or death, people want information and will look for it wherever they can find it. One of the most important and meaningful things you can do for your staff and students is to deliver accurate information about the death in a timely, sensitive manner.

The death of a staff member or student impacts the whole school community. While some students and staff may be more affected than others, the death needs to be acknowledged by the community at large. Of course, there are deaths which affect only a few students or staff members who are acquainted with the person who died. Examples may include a part time staff member, a coach known to a small group of students and staff, a teacher's friend, or a student's relative.

The Crisis Response Team can determine which staff members and students need information about the death and how to present the information accurately and sensitively. It's important to get information about a death to the school community in a timely manner. Even if you cannot provide all the information, tell people as much accurate information as you do know.

Telling Staff

Mr. Jones, a beloved sixth grade teacher at a Catholic school, suffered a heart attack one September, but was recovering nicely and had planned to return to his class after the Christmas holidays. On New Year's Eve, he had a fatal heart attack. His funeral was held several days before teachers returned to class. The principal made an effort to tell a few teachers who were close to Mr. Jones, but others did not find out until they arrived back to school after the vacation. Many of the teachers who were not informed were shocked and upset. They felt disregarded and angry that they had not been able to choose whether or not to attend the funeral of an important member of their community. It created conflict among the staff.

If a school staff member or student dies, inform *all* staff members *as soon as possible.* This includes administrators, support staff, and teachers, as well as custodial and kitchen staff, and bus drivers. Staff can be told by a phone call to their home, a written memo, or at an emergency staff meeting at the earliest possible time (before or after school depending on the time of notification). Crisis Response Team members will need a current updated phone tree with correct phone numbers. If a death occurs during vacations, weekends or breaks, make every effort to let teachers know before they return to school.

If the death impacts a smaller number of staff, such as the death of a sibling of a student, you may choose to inform only teachers and staff members who interact with that person on a regular basis. This can be a challenging task because the team may not know who did or didn't know the person who died. If you can't determine this accurately, tell the whole staff. That way, no one will feel left out. No one appreciates being the last one to find out or being left out of the loop in such a situation. Don't forget to inform staff members who are on vacation, ill, or absent for some other reason. And don't assume you know who cares.

It's not uncommon for some staff members to be resistant to addressing the loss in a public way. They may not want to talk about grief and may feel that students do not need to do so either. Sometimes this is because they have personal loss issues they have not addressed or, it may be that they have incorrect information about what children need following a death. Your modeling of appropriate grief responses and leadership will be a valuable asset to your staff.

If you need to tell a staff member that someone died in their family, make sure that someone in their family or a friend is present. Also, find a private space in which to inform them. Remember to make a plan with the staff member in regards to a substitute.

Telling Students

As adults, we often mistakenly believe we can protect children by withholding information from them. The reality is that children and teenagers need and want the truth as much as adults do. When they don't get it from the adults around them, they will discuss and attempt to piece together information among themselves, in the bathroom, on the playground, on the bus or in the halls. Often information received in these ways is incorrect or embellished and can cause worry and confusion for the students. The bottom line is, students need accurate information about the death as soon as possible. You do not need to give them more information than they request. But you do need to answer their questions honestly. For example, "I don't know," may be a truthful answer to a question about the death.

If the deceased was a staff member who had contact with a limited number of students, such as a part time dance team coach, you may elect to inform only students who were closely involved in that activity and knew the staff member. Similarly, if the deceased was a relative or friend of a student, you may only tell students in a specific classroom or students who are involved with the bereaved. When informing the entire student body about a death, you may want to develop a written statement that teachers can use in the classroom. **Do not** present the information about the death over the Public Address (PA) system. It's impersonal. Every student will have his or her personal reaction to the news. Some will react strongly, while others may not react at all. Sharing the news in the security of the classroom allows students to react, ask questions, talk about the impact of the news, and express thoughts and feelings.

If possible, ask teachers to present the information during first period or home room. If there is more than one teacher or an assisting counselor present, a small group format works well. Allow time for students to share their reactions and feelings about the situation. Students may or may not want to share. When it is their turn to talk, allow them to "pass" if they choose. Teachers are advised to provide a handout on typical grief responses, and to lead a discussion with their students about the death. Allow for questions and discussion. Reassure teachers that they do not need to be concerned if they do not know the answer to a question and that the response "I don't know" in such situations is appropriate.

If you need to tell a student someone has died in his or her family, ensure that a close family member or friend is

Melissa, a third grader, didn't want her classmates to know that her father had died of a heart attack. She did not want to be viewed as different from her peers because she no longer had a father. Her teacher respected her wish and did not tell the class. When she returned to school after being gone for a week, everyone wanted to know where she had been and if she was all right. Because of her grief, she wasn't acting like herself. Other children noticed she cried for no reason, seemed more cranky and had trouble staying focused. Since they did not know what was wrong, they could not help Melissa. Eventually, some of her classmates stayed away from her because they didn't understand.

present to share the news with the student. Children prefer to hear the news of a death from someone they know in a safe, private and familiar setting.

Jane, a fifth grader, was called out of math class and asked to report to the principal's office. She thought she was in trouble but didn't know why. When she arrived in the office, she saw her mother and aunt looking very upset. Her mother told her that her dad had just died in an auto accident. Because she was standing in the middle of the office with staff and other students around, Jane wasn't sure how to respond and felt embarrassed. Later she said she would have preferred to have been told in a place where she felt more safe and free to express her feelings.

Jack, age 9, took a different approach. After talking with his dad, he decided to tell his teacher that his mother had died. Jack's father called the teacher, and with her help, extended an invitation to two of Jack's friends to attend his mom's memorial service. Other students made cards for him and sent a basket of his favorite candy. When Jack returned to school, his classmates were supportive and stood by him when he was having a bad day.

Jessica, a young mother and volunteer in her son Brian's second grade classroom, was found murdered on the sidewalk just one block from his school. Many of the students rode past the spot on their way to school that morning and saw the area cordoned off with yellow police tape. The teachers at the school were reluctant to

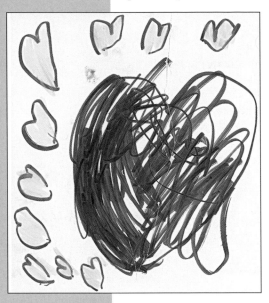

tell the children what had happened. Concerned that the children wouldn't understand, the teachers wanted to protect them from the horrible details. Instead, they chose to inform the parents of the death and asked them to tell their children that evening. The following day children came to school with very different stories about what happened. Some had not been told, while others knew that she died. Some children recounted information they had learned from their parents while others shared what they had heard on the news or had overheard in adult conversations. Many children were afraid. Soon it became clear to the staff that the students needed to be told the same information because they were getting distorted stories from one another. Once the children had correct information, teachers and parents could begin a discussion about safety and other issues that concerned them.

Telling Parents

Parents are part of the grieving community. It is important to inform parents about the situation and what is being shared with their children. A letter sent home with the student, or mailed, or a personal phone call from a staff member is encouraged. It's helpful to have an "information statement" or letter prepared which can be used in such situations *(See Appendix B)*. The letter should include the facts of the death, what was shared with the students, behaviors parents might expect from their children, as well as ways they can support their children. You may also consider scheduling a parent meeting where grief related issues can be discussed and related questions answered. This may be especially needed when the circumstances of the death lead to fears or questions about school safety, about suicide prevention, or other issues impacting the entire community.

Sara, a healthy first grader, went home from school, fell ill unexpectedly, and died the same night in the hospital. Many of the parents at the school panicked when they heard about the death the following day. What had caused this girl to die? Was it something at the school? They had many questions and concerns. To address the situation, the school set up a meeting that night where they informed parents about the death and invited a grief counselor and a public health officer to come discuss the situation. Parents were at first relieved to hear that the cause of the death was not contagious. Then they had an opportunity to ask questions about how they could help their children through the grieving process, and how they could support the grieving family.

Plan Schedules and Activities for the First School Day and Week

In the first few days after a death, students and staff may need time to attend funerals and memorial services, address safety issues, and process their own grief. The Crisis Response Team can facilitate this by adjusting the daily schedule to allow for activities such as a school memorial service, and other opportunities for students to address the death. Staff members may also need to take on added responsibilities for facilitating activities, such as a parent meeting, an after school discussion time, or planning a memorial service.

Typically, students appreciate returning to the routine of their school schedule, but are also helped by having the flexibility to take a break when they need it. Upon returning to school after his father's death, 11-year-old Nathan was glad that the classroom structure was still the same. "I just wanted to think about math and reading and not my dad. It helped me feel normal for a little while and forget about my sadness." Weeks later, it hit him one day in math class how much he missed his father. His teacher allowed him to leave class to go speak with the school counselor. Nathan said he appreciated that his teacher understood the difficulty he was having, and allowed him to do what he needed to do.

Provide Safety Measures and Special Services for Students

After a death, particularly a violent death, students may be wondering how to stay safe and to take care of themselves. In one elementary school, a custodian was killed near the school. Judy, age 8, and other neighborhood children, were afraid to walk to school by themselves because the murderer had not been found. Judy told her mother she was afraid that she would be killed too. In response, the neighborhood mothers set up a rotation system for walking the kids to school until they felt safe to go by themselves.

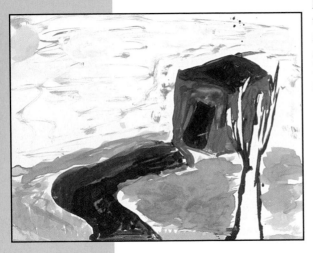

Having a "safe room," where students can go to share feelings, be alone, or talk to others, is extremely important. That space can be located in the main office, counselor or nurse office, an unused classroom or the library. It is important to have someone staff the room for the first few days, as students use it. Providing art materials and books may be helpful to some students. Often, teachers are concerned that a student may just be getting out of work by asking to go to the safe room. In some cases, this may be true. In general, our experience has been that the room is used appropriately by those who need to be there, and is usually not used for lengthy periods of time. Students who are having particular difficulty may benefit from a referral to the school counselor or a community therapist.

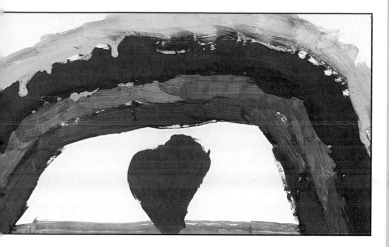

Assign Jobs and Roles to Crisis Response Team Members

"What can I do to help?", concerned staff members often ask after a death. An important part of managing the aftermath of an incident is assigning roles and responsibilities to Crisis Response Team members and to staff who want to help. Some of the team members may already have a designated role, but there is bound to be some juggling of these roles because every situation is different. Here are some safety and health-related tasks which crisis team members and staff can complete following a death. Consider these choices and use what is helpful depending on your situation.

- Plan and arrange for additional counselors and substitute teachers on school grounds.
- Assign a person to respond to media and family requests.
- Set up a plan for additional security on the school grounds.
- Arrange for special or alternative transportation home for the students, if needed.
- Create a "safe room" and arrange for staffing it.
- Notify the superintendent and personnel in other schools about the death.

Here is a checklist of your responsibilities during the school day:

- ☐ Model appropriate leadership and grief response
- ☐ Work with the crisis team regarding the plan and responsibilities
- ☐ Lead staff meeting, discussing the announcement and plan for the day
- ☐ Assist teachers who have asked for help in processing with students
- ☐ Assign staff to the safe room for students
- ☐ Walk the halls, playgrounds, lunchroom; be visible and available
- ☐ Discuss at-risk students and possible interventions
- ☐ Respond to parents who may need support
- ☐ Set up resources for parents
- ☐ Mobilize peer support programs or other school support
- ☐ Plan and lead an after school debriefing for staff
- ☐ Provide support during the school day for any staff who need it
- ☐ Check in with other crisis team members and reassess plans and schedules as necessary
- ☐ Send condolence note to the family

The School Day

After a school community has received news of a death, what happens? How are schedules affected? The following is a general outline and some things to be aware of in the hours and early days after a death.

Staff Briefing and Planning

After the Crisis Response Team has met, a briefing meeting with staff should occur. It is important to have this meeting before the students return to school. All staff who are impacted by the crisis should be included in this meeting. Often this meeting is held for an hour before the school day begins, and staff is notified and requested to attend. At this meeting, be prepared to accomplish the following:

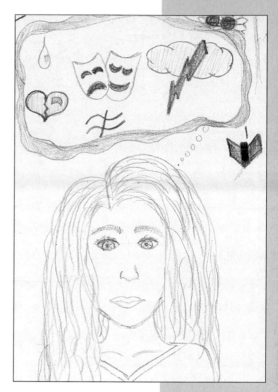

- ☐ Share a written statement and presentation of the circumstances of the death.
- ☐ Prepare teachers to share the information in their homeroom or first period. (It is often helpful for a team of two people to present the information to the students.)
- ☐ Present information about how students grieve and what behaviors might be expected.
- ☐ Review the plan for the school day/week.
  - Stress the need for as routine a day as possible, allowing flexibility (i.e., times for students to talk about the death and its impact on an as needed basis.)
  - Allow for discussion of the plan with staff and adjust as necessary.
- ☐ Address questions and concerns about high risk students with teachers and staff.
- ☐ Discuss the need for substitute teachers for those teachers who need to be away from students for a time because of their own reactions.
- ☐ Identify the location, staffing and use of a "safe room" for students needing additional support throughout the day.
- ☐ Allow time for teachers to talk about their own feelings related to the death/incident.

☐ If applicable, inform teachers of the designated media spokesperson. Advise teachers not to speak with the media or allow them on the school grounds.

☐ Assign a staff person as family liaison.

☐ Announce the schedule for an after school meeting if appropriate to the situation.

Debriefing and Follow-up

At the end of the first school day after a community loss, it is extremely valuable for the staff to reconvene. Staff members may be tired and prefer not to engage in further discussion. But debriefing is an important and necessary part of the grieving process. In addition, debriefing can create a sense of unity and teamwork.

Here are a few things you will want to accomplish in your debriefing:

■ Review the events of the day. Share personal stories, thoughts, feelings.

■ Discuss students you are concerned about and make referrals to the school counselor.

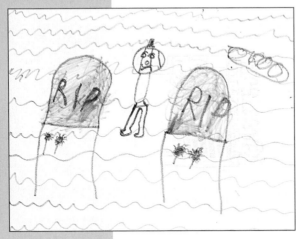

■ Plan for the next few days and weeks.

■ Discuss the memorial service or other memorializing activities.

■ Share resources and information about the staff taking care of themselves physically and emotionally.

Depending on the scope and nature of the death, you may want to set up regular ongoing staff time over the next several weeks to process the impact of the death. Making this a part of a regular schedule will help because these meetings can ensure a healthy grief process for students and staff. Remember, now more than ever, it's important to support one another. No one needs to carry a burden alone.

Student Issues

Modeling and Facilitating Grief

As principal, you will have many opportunities to impact your students after a death occurs. Along with the Crisis Response Team, you will set guidelines for teachers to facilitate classroom discussion and inform students of resources available to them. You will also have opportunities to connect with students during the days and weeks following the death. It may be during an assembly, in your office or in passing in the hall. One of the best things you can do is be a model for grieving. If you acknowledge your own feelings around the loss, and encourage others to do the same, this helps create a safe and open atmosphere for grief.

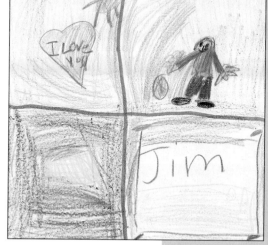

Memorializing the Person Who Died

Another way you can help students and staff is to allow them to play a role in memorializing the person who

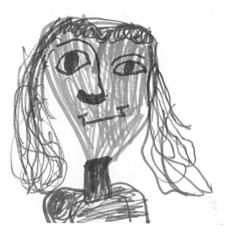

died. Rituals for remembering and memorializing help students and staff begin their healing process. Often students and staff like to plan and participate in a memorial as a way of saying goodbye. For example, students may want to write poetry or share music about the person who died. Other ideas might include:

- writing letters/cards to the family of the deceased
- drawing pictures to remember the person who died
- creating one big card children can sign and send to the family of the deceased

Students may also want to brainstorm ideas for more long-term memorials. Often, what works best is creating a memorial that is personal and reflects the style and personality of the person who died. Here are some examples of memorials:

- After 12-year-old Paul, a soccer player, was killed in a car accident, students and staff at his middle school decided to name a soccer field for him. Later, they held an annual tournament in his name.

- Mr. Thomas, a fifth grade teacher, loved gardening. After his death, the students in his class decided to plant a garden by the entrance of the school.

- Nine-year-old Jamie loved to read. While she was ill with cancer, she spent a lot of time reading in bed. After her death, the students decided to start a library fund in her name and bought new books for all the students to enjoy and remember her.

If you choose not to have a memorial service or activity, you might notice that the students will plan one on their own. When 16-year-old Tiffany died, the school decided not to mention the death or have any sort of memorial. Her friends hung around her locker and placed notes and pictures there. The administration became concerned

When Tommy, a sixth grader, died of cancer, his classmates wanted to remember him in a special way. They left his desk in place and whenever they thought about him, they would write a memory or draw a picture and place it on his desk. All of the students could look at the desk and remember Tommy and how he had impacted their lives. At the end of the school year, the students put all of their pictures and writings together in a book to give to Tommy's family. He remained alive in their memories that year.

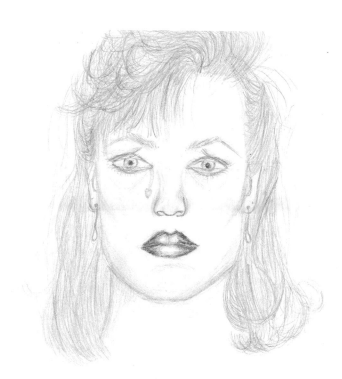

and told the students to disperse. They removed all the belongings from the locker. The students were angry and there was an unfortunate conflict between the students and the administration over the issue.

Your school should have a policy around memorials or other commemorations so that you are prepared *in advance* to deal with such issues. Remember, allowing the students some form of public grief helps them acknowledge the death and the life, and begin the healing. Your policy should include answers to the following questions:

☐ **Will our school provide the opportunity for our community to acknowledge the death of a student or staff member through some kind of memorialization?**

We recommend that you do provide this opportunity, both to acknowledge the life of the person who died, and to be appropriate models for grief and loss.

☐ **What kind of memorialization activities will we sponsor or support?**

Options for activities include sponsoring a community open forum or an evening for parents, students and staff members; holding a school assembly; allowing students to do something commemorative such as planting a tree on school grounds, etc.

☐ **Under what circumstances will we consider memorialization activities? For the death of a staff member or student? For a death by suicide or homicide?**

We strongly urge that whatever policy or precedent the school sets, it should apply to **all** deaths. For example, if you decide that there will be opportunities to acknowledge a student's death publicly and collectively as a school community, you should do **the same thing** for a student who suicides as you would for a basketball player who dies on the court, or a student who is killed in a car accident. When you exclude certain students from being memorialized, you send the message that the student's life was not valued, or that we should sweep suicidal or violent deaths under the rug.

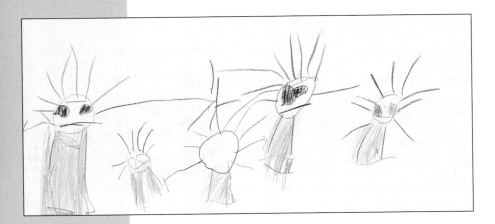

When Andy, a high school sophomore, died by suicide, the school did not want to publicly acknowledge the death. The staff believed that having a remembrance glorified his death and sent a message that they approved of suicide. The administration worried that other children would also kill themselves if the act was talked about at all. This is a common myth. Talking openly about teen suicide does not contribute to its cause. Not talking may actually encourage susceptible youth who already wonder if anyone cares.

If a student in your school dies by suicide, share that information honestly and forthrightly. Many adults are under the mistaken impression that talking about suicide will "put the idea in kids' minds," or increase the likelihood of another attempt. Speaking honestly about this act and the impact it has on others may actually draw out students who are feeling suicidal and enable them to receive help. While many parents are uncomfortable with their children being exposed to the topic of suicide, it is important for children to hear the truth from the adults and educators they trust. When a suicide occurs, the students are talking about it among themselves, whether adults know it or not. It is better to share the factual information and provide help for hurting students rather than try to sweep it under the carpet.

Grief Responses of Students

Everyone grieves differently. Students will react in their own way to the news. Their reactions are impacted by a variety of factors including:

- their age and developmental level
- their relationship, if any, with the deceased
- their previous experience with death
- the support systems available to them
- the modeling of grief responses from those around them
- whether the death was anticipated or unexpected
- the nature of the death

> "I'll never forget how my daughter laughed when I told her her mother died. At first, I was baffled. Then I quickly realized her nervousness."
>
> — John S., father of 14-year-old Kathryn

Of course, not all students will want to talk about the death. You may see students reacting in a variety of ways including being quiet or withdrawn, talking a lot, crying, getting angry, laughing, acting aggressive, looking sad or thoughtful, or any combination of reactions. Each response should be accepted and allowed, as long as it is not harmful to the student or another person. Each response is valid and important to that particular student. Remembering that each person grieves differently, it is important for each student to feel heard and accepted. Remember also that the grief issues will not end at the end of the school day. They can continue into outside activities and home life. Helping parents understand and cope with these issues will be important in the student's life both at school and home.

Here is a list of common responses of the grieving child or teen:

Academic Responses to Grief

- Difficulty focusing or concentrating
- Failing or declining grades
- Incomplete work, or poor quality of work
- Increased absences or reluctance to go to school
- Forgetfulness, memory loss
- Over achievement, trying to be perfect
- Language errors and word finding problems
- Inattentiveness
- Daydreaming

Behavioral Responses to Grief

- Noisy outbursts, disruptive behaviors
- Aggressive behaviors, frequent fighting
- Non-compliance to requests
- Increase in risk-taking or unsafe behaviors
- "Hyperactive-like" behavior
- Isolation or withdrawal
- Regressive behaviors
- Increased need for attention

Emotional Responses to Grief

- Insecurity, issues of abandonment, safety concerns
- Concern about being treated differently from others
- Fear, guilt, anger, rage, regret, sadness, confusion
- "I don't care" attitude
- Change in values, questioning what is important
- Depression, hopelessness, intense sadness
- Regression to times when things felt safer and more in control

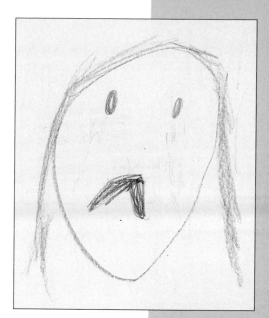

- High need for attention
- Overly sensitive, frequently tearful, irritable
- Appears unaffected by the death
- Preoccupation with death, wanting details
- Recurring thoughts of death or suicide
- A need for checking in on surviving parent(s), sibling(s), friends

Social Responses to Grief

- Withdrawal from friends
- Withdrawal from activities or sports
- Use of drugs or alcohol
- Changes in relationships with teachers and peers
- Changes in family roles (e.g., taking on the role of a deceased parent)
- Wanting to be physically close to safe adults
- Inappropriate sexual behavior/acting out
- Stealing, shoplifting

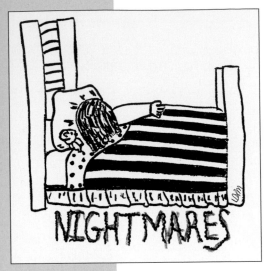

NIGHTMARES

Physical Responses to Grief

- Stomachaches, headaches, heartaches
- Frequent accidents or injuries
- Increased requests to visit the nurse
- Nightmares, dreams or sleep difficulties
- Loss of appetite or increased eating
- Low energy, weakness
- Hives, rashes, itching
- Nausea, or upset stomach
- Increased illnesses, low resistance to colds and flu
- Rapid heartbeat

Spiritual Responses to Grief

- Anger at God
- Questions of "Why me?" and "Why now?"
- Questions about the meaning of life
- Confusion about where the person who died is
- Feelings of abandonment and emptiness
- Doubting or questioning previous beliefs
- Seeing the future as meaninglessness

Identifying Students Who Are At-Risk:

Any student can potentially be at-risk after a death. Communicate with your faculty about observing, listening to and attending to the needs of grieving students. They can help identify those who need a little extra support. Certain kids you may want to pay attention to include those who are:

- directly impacted by the crisis
- not directly impacted by the current crisis but handling a recent tragedy in their own life

- undergoing the stress of accumulated losses (e.g., deaths, divorces, moves, parental unemployment, etc.)
- receiving support for special needs
- dealing with other mental health issues (e.g., depression, eating disorders, behavioral problems, anxiety disorders, etc.)

At-risk behaviors associated with grief may include:

- Aggressiveness
- Truancy or increased absences
- Defiance, non-compliant behavior
- Lack of follow through on assignments
- Falling or failing grades
- Depression
- Suicidal threats or behavior
- Increase in drug or alcohol use
- Increase in risk-taking behaviors

Students who engage in at-risk behavior should be monitored. If the behavior is frequent, and continues over time, or if it is dangerous, refer the student to a counselor for additional support.

Staff Issues

Staff members may also experience emotional, behavioral, social, physical and spiritual responses to a death, particularly if they knew the person who died or if they are intimately involved in counseling or working with grieving students. In addition, staff can be vulnerable to prolonged stress symptoms resulting in:

- Increased absences
- Morale problems
- Performance issues
- Lack of attention to tasks
- Increasing health problems

You can help your staff by checking in with them, providing times and places for them to discuss their grief and to debrief from a day of working with grieving students. Some staff members may need more support than others. Have a list of community resources available in a central location. When possible, allow a staff member to take a day off if necessary.

Dealing with the Media

Sometimes the media is interested in details surrounding a death. If there is a murder, accident, violent death, or if the death was of a prominent person in the school community, members of the media may want to talk to staff or students. James, age 12, found himself in the media spotlight after his dad died in an explosion caused by a bomb placed in his truck. The story of his dad's death was in the news a lot because the murderer turned out to be a jealous friend. In the early days after the death, James' mother had been successful at keeping the media away from her son. However, when he returned to school, several reporters were waiting for him on school grounds to get the "Boy returns to school" story. School personnel escorted the media off school grounds, but the experience was very upsetting to James.

As a principal, it helps to set clear boundaries around media involvement. A written media policy and an assigned media contact is also helpful. Preferably, the media should not be allowed on the school

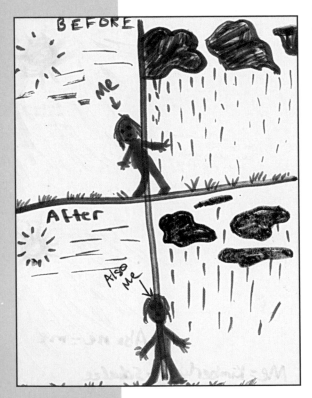

grounds, and the media contact from the school can act as the spokesperson for the school. The contact with the media should be positive and persons should strive to approach the media as an ally rather than the enemy. It is important to let staff know that they should not talk with the media. Student and staff safety and confidentiality is paramount in this regard.

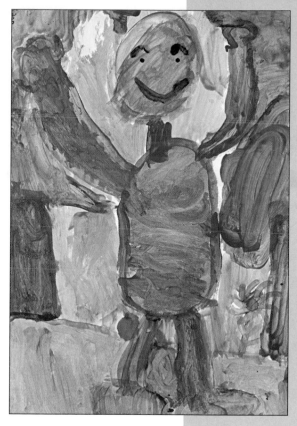

Many students will have difficulty resisting the attention given to them by the media. It is hard for them to resist being interviewed and being in the spotlight. Students often feel torn between not wanting to talk about the crisis and their grief, yet wanting to be important. This is a relevant topic to bring up with students during classroom discussions about what happened.

In incidents where media are likely to be involved, it is important to set clear boundaries, but shutting them out entirely is not a useful or effective strategy. The reality is, their job is to find information and they will do what they can to get it. Try to provide them with accurate, factual information as soon as possible and to have a non-antagonistic relationship. During a crisis, the media can be a valuable resource for community members by sharing information about resource and safety issues. Later on, they may provide information about memorial services or even about the grief process. After one incident in a high school, parents were informed by the media that they could pick up their children across the street from the school at a nearby church.

The Long Term Plan

Grief does not end the day after the funeral. It is not over in a week, a month, or even a year. Grief is an ongoing process which diminishes in intensity but is forever a part of life. The implication for students and faculty is that there will be grief eruptions that are unplanned but powerful. For example, if a shooting has occurred in your school, another shooting somewhere in the country will bring up memories and fears and grief that seemed to be gone.

On the anniversary of the death, students will remember what happened. Acknowledge the date and let students know that you are remembering the person who died on that date. It is important to plan ahead for anticipated events such as the anniversary of the loss or when a similar event occurs. If you follow the media coverage on anniversaries following shooting deaths in Dunsblane, Scotland; Littleton, Colorado and Springfield, Oregon, for example, it is common for teachers, parents and school personnel to make comments like, "We thought this was behind us and that everyone had gotten over it, but the feelings of the kids poured out as if it had happened yesterday." This should not surprise us!

Six Principles of Grieving

When a school community experiences a crisis involving one or more deaths, everyone grieves. We grieve the death of those individuals as well as the inevitable life changes which occur as a result of the loss. While we can prepare ourselves to better manage a crisis, nothing quite prepares us for the grief we experience after a death. And, unfortunately, there are no quick fixes. That's why we offer some basic principles of grieving. These are helpful to keep in mind because they apply to any and all of us who have experienced a death.

1. Grief is a natural reaction to loss.

Grief is a natural reaction to loss. When a person dies, those who are impacted by the death experience emotional and physical reactions. Grief is experienced throughout the life span from infancy to adulthood, although the reaction will vary from person to person.

Grief does not *feel* natural in part because we cannot necessarily control our emotions or other symptoms. The sense of being out of control may be overwhelming or frightening. Grieving is natural, normal, and healthy for bereaved students and adults.

2. Each student's grief experience is unique.

While many theories and models of the grieving process provide a helpful framework of tasks or stages of grieving, the path itself is a lonely, solitary and unique one for every individual. No book, article, or grief therapist can predict or prescribe exactly what a student or an adult will—or should— experience on this path. Those who wish to assist people in grief do so best by walking with them along the path in the role of listener and learner, allowing the griever to teach about his or her unique grief journey.

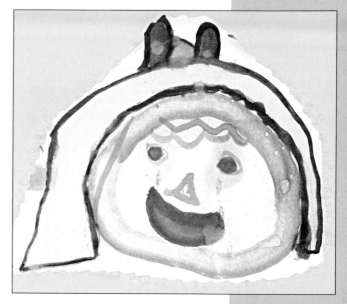

3. There are no "right" and "wrong" ways to grieve.

Coping with a death does not follow a set pattern or set of rules. There is no "right" or "wrong" way to grieve. There are, however, "helpful" choices and behaviors which are constructive, life-affirming actions. Examples might include talking about the death, getting involved in a support group, or creating art work to memorialize the person who died. Other responses are "unhelpful", destructive, or even harmful, causing long-term complications. These might include the use of drugs or alcohol to "numb" the pain, stifling feelings, and avoiding the grief process altogether. The sheer pain of

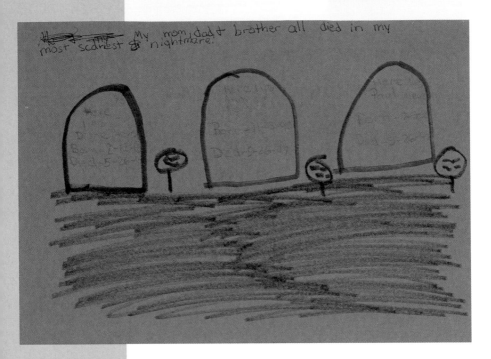

loss often feels "crazy". It can be challenging to decide which thoughts, feelings and actions are helpful, and which are not. Following a death, grieving students get plenty of advice from others about what they should and shouldn't do, feel, think and believe. What is often more helpful than advice is nonjudgmental listening, helping them to sort through the options and alternatives they see.

4. **Every death is unique and will be experienced by your students in different ways.**

Students react differently to the death of a parent, sibling, friend, teacher or principal. Each relationship is unique. Some of the grief literature talks about loss in an almost competitive way as if some losses are worse than others. You may read that the death of a child is the worst loss, or that suicide is the hardest death to get over. Comparisons about which death is the worst are not helpful, and may lead to unrealistic expectations or demands. While a student may speak for himself about how he experienced different losses, one cannot categorically say that any loss is worse, or easier than another. Each person should be respected in *his or her way* of coping with the death.

5. The grieving process is influenced by a multitude of factors.

There are many factors impacting how a student may react to a death. Some of these include:

- the social support systems available to the student (family, school, community, friends)

- the nature of the death and how the student interprets it

- the status of "unfinished business" between the student and the person who died

- the relationship with the deceased

- the emotional and developmental age of the student

- how the community views the death (Stigmatized deaths such as homicides, suicides and AIDS deaths are often looked at very differently than deaths by illness or accident.)

6. Grieving never ends. It is not something the student will "get over."

This is perhaps one of the least understood aspects of grief in our society. Most people are anxious for us to put the loss behind us, to go on, to get over it. When a person dies, the death leaves a vacuum in the lives of those left behind. Life is never the same again. This does not mean life can never again be joyful, or that the experience of loss cannot be transformed into something positive. But grief does not have a magical end. People comment on the pangs of grief 40, 50 or 60 years after a death. For the student at each new developmental level or experience of personal accomplishment, the grieving process will be re-experienced in some new way.

> *"I've had teachers say you've got to go on, you've got to get over this. I just want to shout 'You're wrong! Grief never ends.' I don't care what they say."*
>
> —Philip, 13

Special Concider- ations

Death from Chronic Illness

Death from an illness often evokes issues around one's own health. Children want to share common experiences around the dying process such as hospitalization, medical procedures, emergencies, changes in personality due to an illness, affects of the illness on the relationship, and

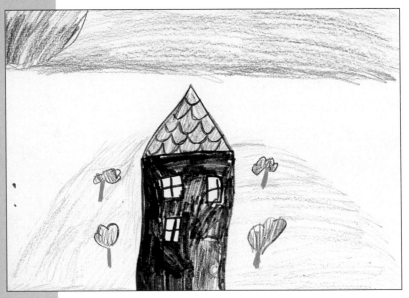

social concerns. Children may feel relieved that the person died because they were no longer in pain.

Children and teens who have a family member die from an illness may experience anticipatory grief. That is to say, they may begin to experience grief responses before the death. They may be tearful or have low energy. They may find it difficult to concentrate. Dealing with a long-term illness can be a fatiguing and emotionally draining experience for a family. It helps if you can keep communication lines open with family members during this time, and be sensitive to concerns that may arise periodically. It is important to remember that a student will probably grieve both during the illness and after the death. The anticipation of the death allows them to say goodbye but there is still grief when the person dies.

Students who have an ill sibling or parent may also feel lonely and neglected due to the fact that there is a lot of attention and energy going toward caring for the dying person.

It has been our experience that students who have had a family member die of AIDS usually only share that the person died, and do not share how that person died, due to the social stigma associated with AIDS deaths. They may fear that if they do share about the death they will be ostracized by the group. Because of their tendency to hold their feelings inside, they may experience more physical symptoms and concerns about their own health. If a student is willing to share that the person died from AIDS, it is helpful to educate other students about the disease.

Chad, age 8, was the only member of his grief support group who had a family member die from AIDS. When asked directly by other children how his mother died, he often chose not to answer or said she died of cancer. One day an adult facilitator in the group shared that his good friend Al had just died of AIDS and that he was very sad. When it was Chad's turn to share, he said for the first time that his mother had died the same way. He was not alone or different any more.

Accidental Death

It was the first day of school after Christmas break. Susan, a fifth grade teacher, headed to work early in the morning to get a jump on the day. As she turned into the parking lot, she was surprised to see a cross made of flowers lying in the driveway. Her thoughts raced. Had something happened during the break? Did a student die? She wondered why she didn't hear anything. Once inside the building, she received a memo from her principal detailing what had happened. An elderly couple crossing the street by their school had been hit by a car. The man died, and his wife was in critical condition. The driver of the car was a parent with two children at the school. The principal asked in his memo that teachers be concerned and sensitive to issues the children might bring up.

Susan came prepared to discuss the matter with her students. Not surprisingly, the children brought up the

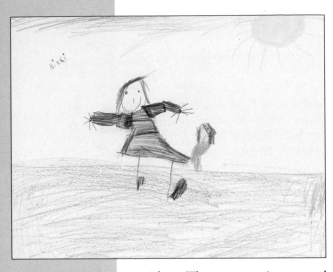

matter first. Some wanted to talk about the elderly couple involved in the accident. One boy said he knew the couple from their church. Another child lived on the same street as the couple. Others were reminded of their own losses. A boy spoke about the death of his mother in a motorcycle accident. The conversation turned to issues of safety when a student shared new information about the accident. He said that the parent driving had been distracted by a child in a car seat and turned around to attend to the situation when the accident occurred. The children asked if there was anything that could be done to prevent such an accident. They talked about the importance of being well-behaved passengers in the car and on the school bus so as not to distract the driver.

Many important topics were covered on this day, and students felt safe discussing it with their teacher and each other. The conversations, though not prolonged, gave students an opportunity to discuss what was on their minds.

Suicide, Homicide and Other Stigmatized Deaths

After her son died by suicide, Lydia Moore often said to children and adults who had learned about the death: "You're probably wondering what in the world to say to me." This was a very helpful ice-breaker. The truth is, people often don't know what to say. Unfortunately, and sometimes without realizing it, people may also judge those who die by a death such as AIDS, suicide or murder. Their surviving family members are often judged harshly as well. In general, people do not know what to say or how to be around survivors of stigmatized deaths. Because of their discomfort, friends and family of the griever will stay away, not offering the same level of support they would if the death were from a car accident, cancer or other disease. This is very hard on the grieving student and family, who often have little or no support after such a death. Aside from the stigma, family members also often feel ashamed or guilty. They wonder if they could have prevented the death. All of these factors play a part in how people are impacted by stigmatized deaths.

One way to help students and adults who experience this kind of loss is to talk with them about how the person died, using the appropriate words such as "killed," "murdered," "shot," "hung," or "suicided." Although using these words with your students may be difficult, it is important for them to hear the truth from caring adults rather than from the evening news, or from other students on the school grounds.

Death by Suicide

Death by suicide often evokes issues of abandonment, shame, and social stigma. Students impacted by a suicide need to understand that they are not alone, to learn how to manage the anxiety that may result from the suicide, and to talk about why a person suicides. Although not quite as extreme as they once were, negative views of suicide persist in our language and our funeral practices. People say a person "commits" suicide or "takes his life." Usually when we speak of "committing" acts, we are referring to crimes or sins. People who die by suicide are often not treated with the same honor or respect as those who die by other means. Sometimes, there is no memorial service or obituary. As a result, people don't get a chance to say goodbye to the person who died.

School personnel are often afraid to recognize a suicide death for fear of the "contagion effect." They worry that if they talk about a suicide death, others will kill themselves or that it will glorify the death. We believe that a suicide death should be treated in the same manner as any other type of death. It is extremely rare for a suicide to be followed by another, and is more likely to occur when the first suicide is not treated with respect, compassion and peer prevention efforts.

In the case of a death by suicide, the surviving family members are often confused as to why the person died. They may experience guilt over not having prevented the death, or they may be extremely angry at the deceased

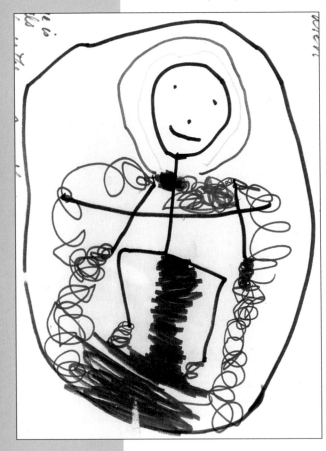

for having taken his or her own life. Students impacted by a suicide may have more chaotic energy or physical complaints, especially stomachaches. They often avoid the area where the death occurred, and fear being alone. For some students there is a sense of relief at the death because of the tension or anxiety surrounding the deceased. If the parent was mentally ill or affected by drugs or alcohol, their behavior may have been embarrassing or hard for the student to understand and handle. The death releases them from the concern.

Discussion about the disease in the brain and the chemical imbalances persons experience helps students to understand a suicide death.

Because deaths by suicide are often judged harshly by our society, children and teens impacted by a suicide frequently do not want others to know how the person died although they usually find out. Mary, age 12, said she felt like a "freak" after her father's suicide. One 16-year-old reported that while standing at her locker between classes in the crowded hallway another student yelled at her, "No wonder your mother blew her brains out! I would too if I had a daughter like you!"

Watch for signs that the student is being teased or avoided by other students, and make an extra effort to provide support and understanding. Frequently children and teens who are acting out and have had a parent or sibling die by suicide are experiencing teasing from others.

Allow for a memorial to remember the person who died. The implementation of a suicide prevention curriculum is helpful for educating children and teens about depression, mental illness, warning signs and ways to get help.

Murder or Violent Death

When she was nine, Marianne's father died of a gunshot wound to the heart. He had been walking on a road through a clear cut area near a hunting party when he was shot. The shooter was never found, and the family never really knew if the death was an accident or a murder. Like many children who are impacted by violent death, Marianne was afraid that the person might come and kill her.

A few years after her father's death, a man with a hunting rifle was spotted by police near her elementary school. In response, the school "locked down" the building. Children were not permitted to leave the building, use the bathrooms, or call parents. They also had no meals. The shades were drawn in the classrooms, and children were asked to play games quietly and to wait until the end of the school day or until their parents came to pick them up. At one point, Marianne took refuge under her desk because she felt afraid and was crying. She told her mom later that she worried that the man who killed her dad would come and kill her.

Watching the news later that night, Marianne and her sister Naomi learned that the man with the rifle had not been found. To add to their stress, they also heard a story about the number of people killed in hunting accidents. Neither girl wanted to go back to school the next day. They were afraid.

Anne had several conversations with the vice principal at her school. She was frustrated by their apparent inability to understand the fear her daughters had about their safety. "He told me I was being really ridiculous and that I should just trust that the school had it under control," Anne said. "They also didn't understand that kids can be fearful long after the death. They seemed to think death happens, you bury the person and go on. But with kids, it's different."

Some thing that scares me is when I think of my step dad and the fact that he hated me and he killed my mom when she was lieing in bed. and that he could have killed me

I hated him. well I forgive him he had a lot of ange

As a parent, Anne also felt frustrated that there hadn't been any communication on the day of the incident between school administrators and parents. In fact, the only word about the incident came in the form of a letter mailed to parents three weeks later. There was no discussion about safety procedures or plans that were employed by the school to address the event. Anne said

she would have liked more information and the security
of knowing that the school had a plan.

> *"When you've had something violent happen to you, you
> never use the word "never" because you know it can happen,"
> said Anne, a parent at an elementary sxhool. "Schools have fire
> drill plans. Why not have another plan in place for crises?"*

Death from a murder often evokes issues around safety,
loss of control, fear, rage, and powerlessness. There may
also be public humiliation from the media attention and
on-going legal investigations. Children need to share
their fears and feelings of wanting revenge, to receive
assistance in managing the anxiety that may result from
their issues, and to be given choices for accessing their
sense of control and power.

If children witness a violent death, they may have
symptoms of trauma and caregivers will need
information on these symptoms and how to respond.
Those who experience a death by homicide are often
judged negatively by others. Sometimes others, in an
effort to protect themselves from the possibility that a
murder could happen to someone they love, believe that
the murdered one's family must have, in some way,
contributed to the event—that "bad things only happen
to bad people." Obviously this attitude alienates those
who are impacted by a homicide.

Other factors that may make coping more difficult
after a homicide are the impact of the media and trial. If
the murderer is caught, there is someone to be angry
with, but families seldom feel, whatever the verdict, that
justice is done. Even if the accused is found guilty and
sentenced to life in prison, they get to eat, breathe and
sleep, while the loved one is dead. If no one is ever
caught, many children and teens express fear that the
person will come and harm them.

After a sudden and violent death the students may feel
frightened, and concerned about their own safety and the
safety of those around them. Teachers may see increased
absences of students, and may notice students' fear of

getting to and from school, and concern on the play ground. There may be an increase in aggressive behavior and violent play. These students tend to become withdrawn from their peers.

As principal, you need to meet with teachers and counselors to discuss and implement plans for safety. For example, you may want to have more adults out at recess, or have a parent walk with the children to school. Reassure the students that school is as safe as possible.

You may also want to review with your staff some of the issues that might come up for students who have been traumatized. For example, students who have had a family member or friend murdered may show signs of Post Traumatic Stress Disorder. These include:

- persistent nightmares or flashbacks relating to the trauma

- excessive fears

- flat or depressed affect

- being easily startled

- persistently avoiding places or events or people associated with the trauma

Some students may need to be referred to counseling for help. It is not uncommon that these students have many more fears. One six-year-old used to lie down on the bus seat every time she went past the apartment complex where her father's murderer had lived. Even though he was in prison for life, she was still concerned that he would see her and come to kill her as well. They often do not feel safe being outside in the open and like to stay near adults for safety. Providing them with choices about what feels safe to them is important. It is also helpful to allow them a place to vent feelings of anger, rage or revenge. Allow the student to talk about the death if they want. Because the story is usually not pleasant, most people will not want to hear the story again but it is important for the student to continue to share the story as a way of healing.

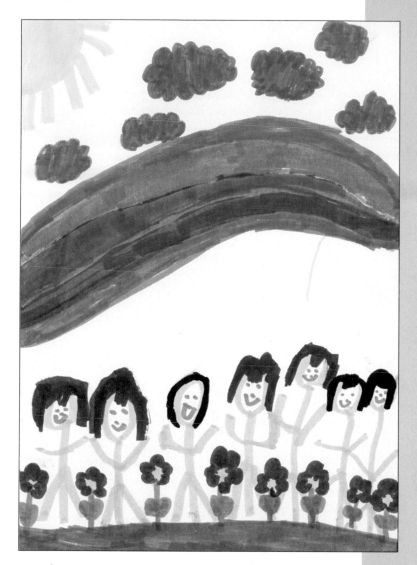

In the unique circumstance that there is a violent death on school grounds, be aware that the school will be overwhelmed by police, outside experts and media. This is a completely different scenario and is beyond the scope of this book. To address a potential crisis of this magnitude, it may be helpful to coordinate with other schools in adopting a district-wide policy on how to handle such events.

Conclusion

As a principal, you have a chance to be a role model for grieving students, staff and parents in your school community. Don't miss out on this opportunity. The things you say and do during a traumatic time have great impact and will be remembered. After one teenage student's father died of a heart attack, her principal took a risk and shared his experience after the death of his father when he was in college. Several years later, the student recalled how hearing his words helped her to feel less alone, and how she was encouraged to learn that despite this loss, he'd grown up and turned out okay. In one rural high school, another principal made a difference when she chose to allow a memorial service for a student who died by suicide. The principal took time to share with students and parents that memorializing a life was not an invitation or affirmation of suicide, but rather an opportunity to grieve the loss of an important member of a school community. With the help of counselors and community resources, the principal also spent time educating the community about suicide and in particular about warning signs as well as the stigma associated with this type of death.

Even if you have never had a personal experience with a death, you have an ability to be an empathic listener and create a safe environment for grieving to occur among students and staff in the school. It may mean discussing some difficult topics, planning ahead, making unpopular decisions and being real about your concerns and feelings. In short, it requires strong leadership, bravery and compassion. Although being supportive may inflict some short-term discomfort for you and others, in the long run students, faculty and parents will be appreciative. You can count on it.

Appendices

Appendix A:

Sample Scripts for Classroom Announcements

- *Share facts of the death*
  Who, What, Where, When, How

- **Accident or general death:**

  I have some very sad news to share today. Janie Smith, a third grader in Mrs. Felts class, was hit by a car while she was waiting for the bus in front of her house yesterday morning. She died at the hospital last night.

  I am feeling pretty sad and would like to take some time to talk about how you are, and answer any questions you might have.

- **Suicide:**

  I would like to share some very sad news with you. Mr. Jones died yesterday at his home. He killed himself by hanging. I know that there will be lots of questions about his suicide and why he did it. Suicide is a very hard death to understand, there are all kinds of questions, the most frequent is "why." We can all talk about it and can answer some of the questions.

- **Violent Death:**

  I have something sad to share with you. Jane Jones, a student who attends our school, has been missing for two days. The police found her body last night in the field behind her house. She had been shot in the head. The police are considering the death a homicide. They have arrested her boyfriend and charged him with murder. When someone is murdered it is very scary for all of us. We will be providing an opportunity for you to talk about the death, share your concerns and fears and answer questions.

Appendix B:

Sample letter to parents after a death

Dear Parent,

A very sad thing has happened in our school community. This weekend, one of our staff, Mr. Smith, a fifth grade teacher and our baseball coach, was hit by a car on his way home from the beach and he was killed. According to his family, a car crossed over into his lane and hit his car head on. He died at the scene of the accident. We are all profoundly saddened by his death.

We have shared this information with your children today and had discussions with all the students in their homeroom. Bereavement counselors, teachers and other support staff have been, and will continue to be, available to students, teachers and parents. Please contact the school if you have any questions or concerns.

As a parent, you may want to talk to your child about death because it impacts each person in different ways. How children will react will depend on the relationship they had with the person who died, their age, and their prior experience with death.

Your child may:

- appear unaffected
- ask questions about the death repeatedly
- be angry or aggressive
- be withdrawn or moody
- be sad or depressed
- become afraid
- have difficulty sleeping or eating

We suggestion that you listen to your children. If they want to talk, answer their questions simply, honestly and be prepared to answer the same questions repeatedly.

(optional) A Parent Informational Night is planned for (date, time and place). At that time, we can talk further about how to help children in grief.

Our thoughts are with (family name).

Sincerely,

Sample letter to parents after a suicide death

Dear Parent,

I have very sad news to share with you. We learned last night that John Smith, a senior in our high school, died by suicide. According to police reports, he shot himself in the woods behind his home. We have shared this information with all of the students in their first period class this morning. We hope that you will be able to talk with your son or daughter about the death.

Suicide is a difficult death for most people to understand and accept because it raises many unanswerable questions. We can never really know why a person kills himself. There can be a variety of factors that lead to an individual's suicide death. Sometimes students, especially John's friends, may wonder if they could have prevented the death. Others may feel that it was somehow their fault. It's important that students have an opportunity to communicate about these concerns and receive help if they need it.

Counselors, teachers and other staff have been and will continue to be available for the students, parents, and teachers to talk about thoughts, feelings and concerns. Please contact us at the school if you have any questions or concerns.

A meeting will be held Tuesday evening at 7:00 p.m. at the school. It is open to parents, students and staff. A bereavement counselor will be presenting information on the suicide issues including symptoms to watch for and prevention efforts. Please plan to attend.

Our thoughts are with the Smith family as they deal with their son's death.

Sincerely,

Sample letter to parents after a violent death

Dear Parent,

I have very sad news to share. We have learned that John Smith, the parent of one of our students, was found murdered in his home last night. The police informed us that a neighbor of the family has been arrested and charged with Mr. Smith's death. However, the death is still under investigation. We shared this information with all of the students in their homeroom classes this morning. We hope that you will be able to talk with your son or daughter about the death. The children will probably have many questions about the death. Honest direct answers are always best.

A violent death may cause a variety of reactions in your child. Many children become afraid that they or someone they love may also be killed. Your child may not want to leave you or come to school. We hope that you will be able to provide messages of safety for them. We have planned some follow up activities to help deal with the fears and provide a measure of safety for the students.

You may notice news reporters around the school. We have asked them to respect the privacy of the students and staff. You do not need to respond to them if you do not want to. We will not allow your children to be interviewed.

Bereavement counselors, teachers and other staff have been and will continue to be available for the students, parents, and teachers. Please contact us at the school if you have questions or concerns.

A meeting will be held Tuesday evening at 7:00 p.m. in the school cafeteria. It is open to parents, students and staff. A bereavement counselor will present information on violent death issues including common grief responses for your child and how you can help. Please plan to attend.

Our thoughts are with the Smith family as they deal with their father's death.

Sincerely,

Also by The Dougy Center for Grieving Children

More in our Guidebook Series:

Helping Children Cope with Death provides a comprehensive, easy-to-read overview of issues facing grieving children, and how others can help. Based on The Dougy Center's work with children, teens and families, this guidebook contains information on a child's understanding of death, developmental issues, how to explain death to children, what helps and what doesn't, how to know when to get professional help, and much more. For parents, teachers, social workers, counselors, youth workers or anyone who knows a grieving child and wants to help. (#534) $9.95

Helping Teens Cope with Death—Adolescence is a period of profound changes. When a teen also deals with a major loss, those developmental changes and the turmoil they create can be compounded. Learn how a death of a loved one can impact a teen and how to help. This practical guide explains common grief reactions of teenagers, specific challenges grieving teens face, advice from parents to parents on supporting an adolescent, when to seek professional help, and much more. An invaluable resource for anyone wanting to support a grieving teen—taken directly from what teens have taught us about supporting them. (#535) $9.95

Helping the Grieving Student: A Guide for Teachers is written specifically to address issues that arise in the classroom after a death impacts a student, a classroom or a school. This guidebook provides teachers of elementary through high school aged students with a complete understanding of how to help children and teens impacted by death. Included are practical, usable tips and step-by-step information on what to say and do and what not to say and do. Information on developmental issues affecting different age groups of grieving students and specific activities for use in the classroom are also included. (#536) $9.95

35 Ways to Help a Grieving Child—If you know a child who has experienced the death of a mother, father, caregiver, sister, brother or friend, you may have wondered how you can help. In this guidebook, we've gathered together the most important stuff we've learned from the grieving children and teens who have come to The Dougy Center since 1982. These 35 practical suggestions for helping grieving children are particularly helpful to those who have recently experienced the death of a family member or friend as they cope with the new tasks of mourning. (#546) $9.95

What About the Kids? Understanding Their Needs in Funeral Planning and Services–By adulthood, most of us have known someone who died and have attended a funeral. But what is a funeral like for a child or teenager who unexpectedly loses a parent, sibling, grandparent or friend? And how do children say goodbye? This guidebook was developed by The Dougy Center to help parents and caregivers support children before, during and after a funeral or memorial service. We've gathered practical suggestions and ideas about what kids want and need from funerals. *What About the Kids?* suggests options for involving children and teens in memorial services and how to explain terms such as burial and cremation to children. Includes suggestions from children and teens on what was helpful and what wasn't at funerals they attended. (#547) $9.95

For recent additions to our guidebook series, please give us a call: 503•775•5683 or check our website: www.dougy.org.

Additional Resources Available from The Dougy Center

Books:

Help For the Hard Times: Getting Through Loss, Earl Hipp. Hazelden, Center City, MN

This attractively illustrated guide takes the teen reader on a journey called grief with a map to help them find their way. (#538) $15.00

Waving Goodbye: An Activity Manual for Children in Grief—Packed with over 45 activities to use with children and teens in peer-to-peer grief support groups, the manual is an essential resource for anyone working with grieving children. The activities, generated from The Dougy Center and network programs across the United States, are organized by category: feelings, memorializing, healing, family, rituals and special days, closure and saying goodbye and more. (#502) $35.00

The above resources can be ordered through:

The Dougy Center
PO Box 86852
Portland, OR 97286

503•775•5683
FAX: 503•777•3097

Website: www.dougy.org

What is The Dougy Center?

The mission of The Dougy Center is to provide loving support in a safe place where children, teens and their families who are grieving a death can share their experience as they move through their healing process. Through our National Center for Grieving Children and Families, we also provide support and training locally, nationally and internationally to individuals and organizations seeking to assist children and teens in grief.

The Dougy Center serves children and teens ages 3-19 who have experienced the death of a parent or sibling (or, in the teen groups, a friend), to accident, illness, suicide or murder. The support groups are coordinated by professional staff and trained volunteers. In addition, the parents (or caregivers) of the youth participate in support groups to address their needs and the issues of raising children following a traumatic loss.

When The Dougy Center was established in 1982, it was the first grief peer support program of its kind in the country. In response to numerous requests for information about our program, The Dougy Center developed trainings and publications to help other communities establish centers for grieving children and families. Through our National Center for Grieving Children, The Dougy Center has trained individuals and groups throughout the world, and publishes a National Directory of Children's Grief Services, updated annually.

The Dougy Center is a 501(c)3 nonprofit organization

and raises its entire budget through contributions from individuals, businesses and foundations. We receive no government funding, or third party payments. Participating families may contribute to the program, but there is no fee for service. While families receiving services contribute what they can, many do not have the financial resources to donate. Since the Center will never turn a family away because of their inability to contribute, we are totally reliant on private support from our friends in the community.

How can I support The Dougy Center or get additional information about your programs?

Contributions to The Dougy Center are tax-deductible to the full extent allowable under IRS guidelines. Your gift can be made out to The Dougy Center and mailed to us at the address below.

You can receive additional information about:

- Other guidebooks available from The Dougy Center

- Videos and other resource materials available from The Dougy Center

- Training on developing a children's grief center in your area

- The National Summer Institute held annually at The Dougy Center on developing a children's grief center in your area

- How to schedule a training or presentation in your area

- Supporting The Dougy Center and its local and national programs to assist grieving children through a will or bequest

Write, call, fax, or E-mail:

The Dougy Center
PO Box 86852
Portland, OR 97286

503•775•5683
FAX: 503•777•3097

E-mail: help@dougy.org
Website: www.dougy.org

Contributors to the Guidebook include The Dougy Center staff:

Amy R. Barrett, M.S.,
Director of Children's Grief Services/Writing & Editing

Joan Schweizer Hoff, M.A.,
Associate Director/Writing & Editing

Donna L. Schuurman, Ed.D.,
Executive Director/Writing & Editing

Donald W. Spencer, M.Div., M.Ed., M.Coun.Psy.,
Director of Family Services/Editing

Kerry Walls, M.A.,
Director of Educational Outreach/Editing & Project Management

Stephen Guntli, CFRE,
Director of Planning & Development/Editing

Berjé A. Barrow,
Director N/NE Program /Writing & Editing

Kellie Campbell,
Executive Assistant/Editing

Cole Struhar,
Program/Network Assistant

Sharrin Campbell,
Administrative Assistant

Pat Madison,
Office Administrator

Cover Art/Inside Art:
Provided by children from The Dougy Center

Design:
Fran Fitzsimon/Fitzsimon GRAFIX

When death impacts your school

The Dougy Center
could not exist without the generous contributions of
hundreds of volunteers
who give of their time, boundless energy,
unflagging enthusiasm and matchless dedication.

We thank them for accompanying
the children, teens and adults
who come to The Dougy Center
in their grief journey.

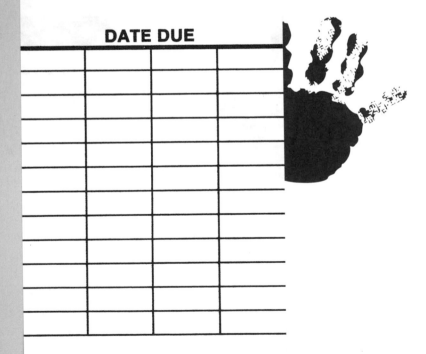

DATE DUE